THE EASY GUIDE
to Preparing for a Healthy Pregnancy

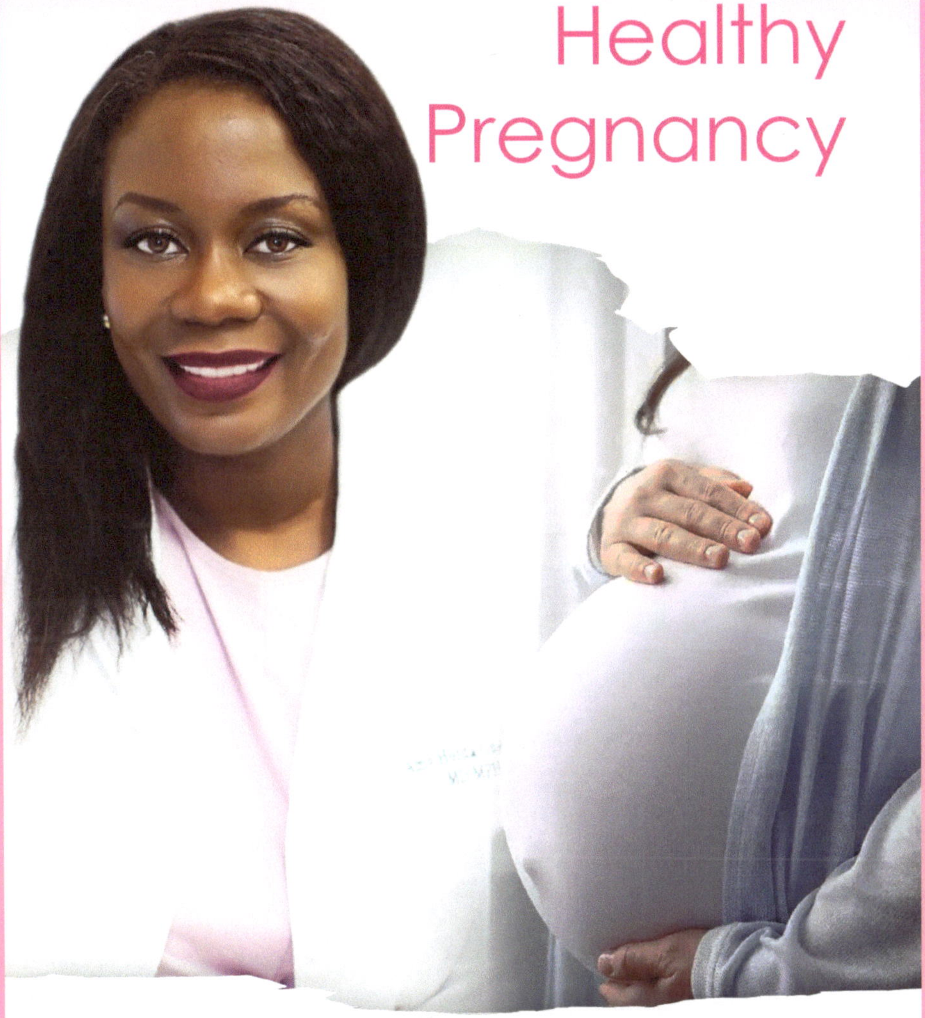

By Top American OBGYN
Dr Amy Holda Gueye-Weinstein

DR. HOLDA GUEYE

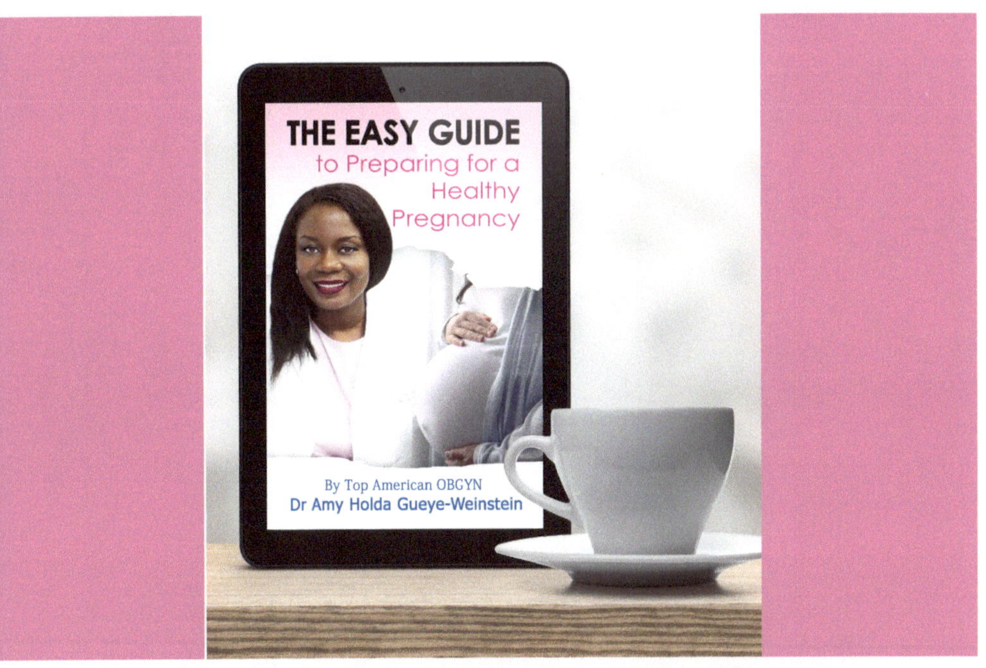

DR. HOLDA GUEYE-WEINSTEIN
Board Certified Top OBGYN

Dr. Gueye-Weinstein is a highly respected and renowned OBGYN, board-certified by the American Board of Obstetrics and Gynecology. She completed her rigorous training at Johns Hopkins, one of the most prestigious medical institutions in the world. Her expertise in the field of OBGYN has earned her recognition as one of the top doctors in both the United States and internationally. Dr. Gueye-Weinstein is sought after as a tertiary referral for second opinions and challenging cases. What sets Dr. Gueye-Weinstein apart is not just her exceptional medical skills, but also her warmth, compassion, and unmatched bedside manner. Patients describe her as an attentive listener who genuinely cares about their overall well-being. She aims to fully understand her patients' health picture, allowing her to provide optimal outcomes tailored to each individual.

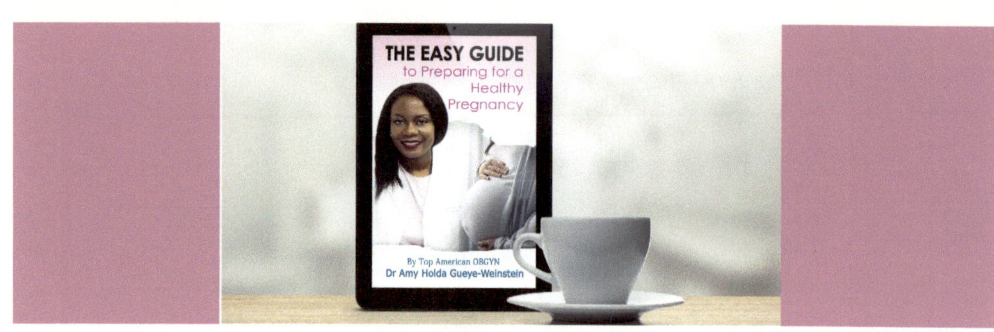

(continued)

In addition to her extensive medical training, Dr. Gueye-Weinstein has pursued further education in herbal medicine. She understands the importance of integrating traditional medicine with functional medicine, respecting both approaches while advocating for a holistic, root cause-oriented approach to medical care.

Dr. Gueye-Weinstein is not only a dedicated physician but also a mother, an author, and the founder of the HALFA non-profit organization, which has been saving the lives of women in Africa since 2012. She is a TEDx speaker, giving a groundbreaking talk on how our emotions can lead us to well-being or disease. Her commitment to the field has earned her numerous awards and recognition. Dr. Gueye has also conducted research at the National Cancer Institute on malaria and breast cancer genomics.

Dr. Gueye-Weinstein's passion for global health led her to pioneer the "see and treat" cervical dysplasia method used in resource-poor settings worldwide. This groundbreaking project was initiated while she was still in medical school, demonstrating her dedication to making a significant impact.

Dr. Gueye-Weinstein's dedication, diverse skill set, and comprehensive approach to healthcare make her a leading figure in the field of OBGYN. Patients can expect exceptional, personalized care from a physician who truly goes above and beyond for her patient's well-being and overall health.

CONTENTS

CONTENTS

INTRODUCTION

Congratulations!
You have decided that a journey as a mother is in your future. The fact that you also picked up a book like this one to prepare for it should be applauded and celebrated. Your decision to be proactive about your health and the pregnancy process will ensure a much higher likelihood of success, peace of mind, and health for you and your future baby.

This guide can be used alone but becomes even more powerful when used in conjunction with your obstetrician. You can bring up the issues at hand that pertain to you and open the floor for an informed discussion where your questions can be directed and knowledgeable, ensuring the best outcomes for you.

I encourage you to choose a doctor who does not make you feel rushed through the visit, answers all your questions, and, most importantly, with whom you feel heard, seen, and understood. Beware of doctors who dismiss your symptoms, make assumptions about who you are and your lifestyle, or are difficult to reach in times of need. Pregnancy is a delicate time where you need to gather around you a solid, caring, compassionate, and competent team that will carry you through. It really does take a village, and later in this book, I will show you how to get this village together.

(Continued)

The choices you will make in the months preceding your pregnancy and your state of health will become one of the most important determinants of your outcomes. This is the perfect time to
make the necessary changes and take the necessary steps to optimize these outcomes.

This book will cover everything you need to know to get ahead of this beautiful journey you are about to embark on.

Congratulations again, and I am honored to walk with you on this journey.

Dr. Amy Holda Gueye-Weinstein
MD, MPH, FACOG

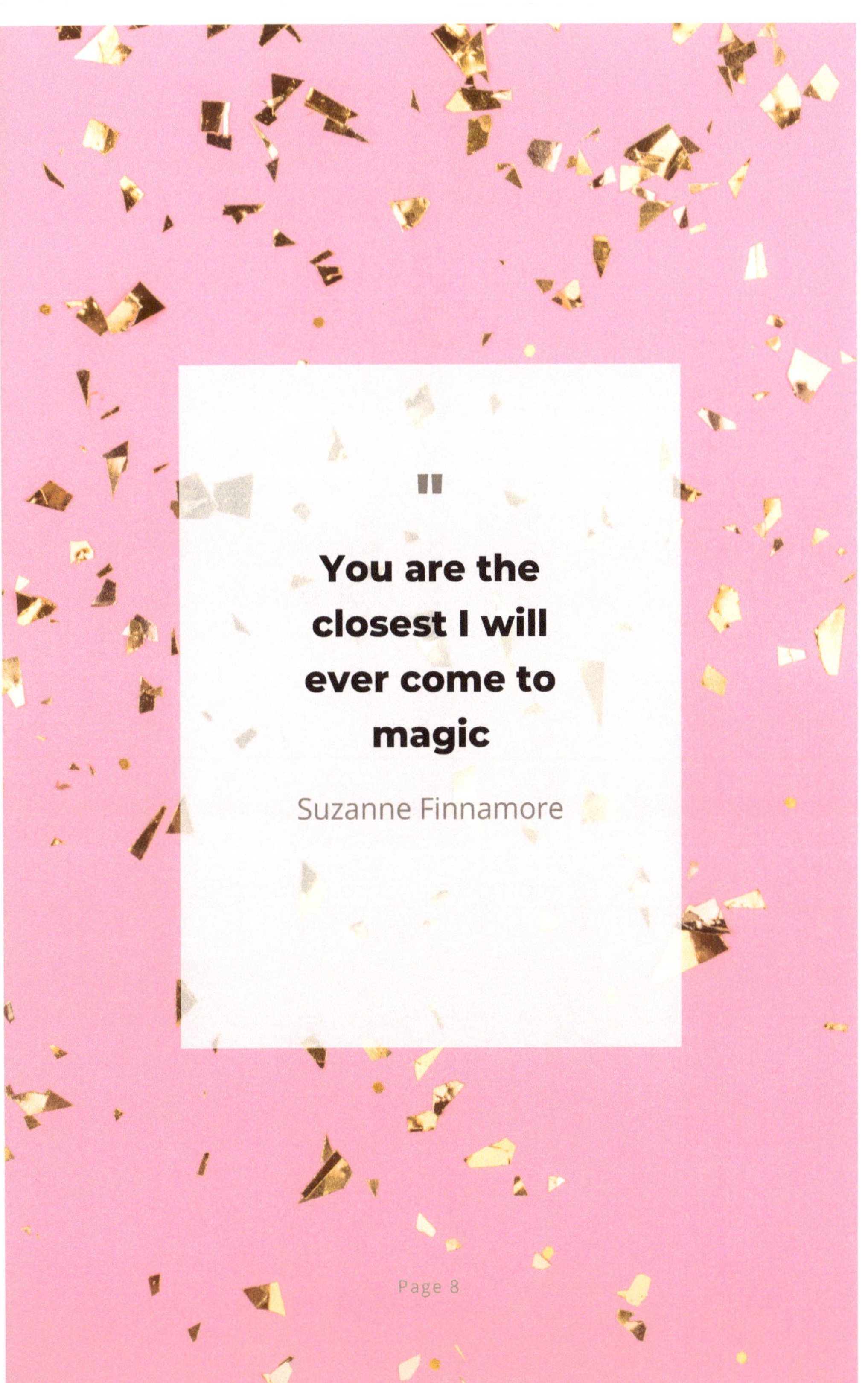
"
You are the
closest I will
ever come to
magic

Suzanne Finnamore

CHAPTER 01

STABILIZING ACTIVE MEDICAL CONDITIONS BEFORE PREGNANCY

Some medical problems can worsen during pregnancy while others improve or stay the same. If you begin your pregnancy at the poor end of the spectrum, some can be very difficult to stabilize due to our limited access to safe treatments. If you still need to get your general wellness and well-woman checkups with your gynecologist, ensure this is completed before you start trying to conceive. Many women who previously thought they were healthy can uncover problems with their blood sugars, cholesterol, blood pressure, and more, from this simple, life-saving visit. These should be updated every year.

If you have known medical problems, it will be important to stabilize them before you begin conception. Let your managing provider know that you plan to conceive soon. This should alert them to review your medications and take you off any that may be dangerous for the developing fetus. You can, and should always, ask your OBGYN to give their input on the medication changes in preparation for pregnancy. Below we will review the most common health conditions and how they can affect pregnancy.

HYPERTENSION (HIGH B LOOD PRESSURE)

High blood pressure can be exacerbated by pregnancy because blood cell production increases in the body to support the growth and nourishment of the fetus. This can cause more pressure on the heart and kidneys leading to kidney and heart diseases. Hypertension also increases the risk of preeclampsia, preterm birth, and Caesarean section.

 Hypertension affects the fetus by limiting blood supply to the placenta. This results in low oxygen and nutrient supply to the fetus, eventually leading to fetal growth restriction.

Hypertension, if left untreated or uncontrolled, can lead to pre-eclampsia. Pre-eclampsia is a condition of pregnancy characterized by high blood pressure with a significant amount of protein leaking out into the urine, which we call proteinuria. Pre-eclampsia needs immediate management because it can lead to eclampsia: seizures and high blood pressure characterize the classical presentation of eclampsia and this is a medical emergency.

 If you are planning a pregnancy and you have hypertension, you should see your primary care provider to manage and control your blood pressure levels. Here are some lifestyle modifications that can directly improve your blood pressure before pregnancy

TIPS:

- Decrease your sodium intake (1500 mg is the daily recommended amount for those with hypertension)
- Manage your Stress response.
- Start moving more. Make sure that you have an enjoyable exercise routine that you perform for at least 30 minutes each day.
- Improve your diet. Avoid processed foods, minimize flour and refined sugars, and increase whole foods.
- Ensure that you are drinking at least 2L of water a day or more

TYPE 2 DIABETES

Type-2 diabetes, if left untreated or uncontrolled, will result in diverse complications for both mother and fetus during pregnancy. Here are a few problems that a diabetic patient can face during pregnancy:

- High blood pressure
- Pre-eclampsia
- Eclampsia
- Too much amniotic fluid (polyhydramnios)
- Early Labor and delivery (Preterm labor/delivery)
- Stillbirth
- Increased Risk of Cesarean Section

The fetus of a diabetic mother can face the following:

- Baby is too large (Macrosomia)
- Breathing problems
- Low glucose level
- Jaundice (yellowing of the skin)

These mentioned complications can be prevented by keeping your glucose levels in the normal range, before and during pregnancy. Your hemoglobin A1C is a great marker for how your overall blood sugar control has been over the preceding 3 months and a number less than 6 is good, less than 5.7 is ideal.

TIPS:

- Discuss helpful supplements such as Berberine 500 mg three times a day with your doctor as a way to help manage your blood sugar metabolism alongside any necessary prescriptions and lifestyle modifications prior to conceiving.

THYROID DISEASE

Thyroid disease can interfere with the normal process of ovulation required for conception. However, if you are pregnant, thyroid disease can cause many complications including miscarriage, pre-eclampsia, premature birth, and low birth weight. Hypothyroidism during pregnancy results in defective psychomotor development of the fetus. Therefore, proper treatment of thyroid disease, before and during pregnancy is advised.

Your thyroid function is measured with two blood tests. One is called TSH (Thyroid Stimulating Hormone) and the second is called T4. Some providers will also order T3 and rT3

LUPUS

Lupus is an autoimmune disease that affects multiple organs and systems in the body. Lupus is notorious for causing pregnancy loss or miscarriage. It can also result in complications like pre-eclampsia, fetal growth restriction, preterm birth, and stillbirth. Patients with lupus systemic erythematosus are advised to get full treatment and regression of the disease before getting pregnant.

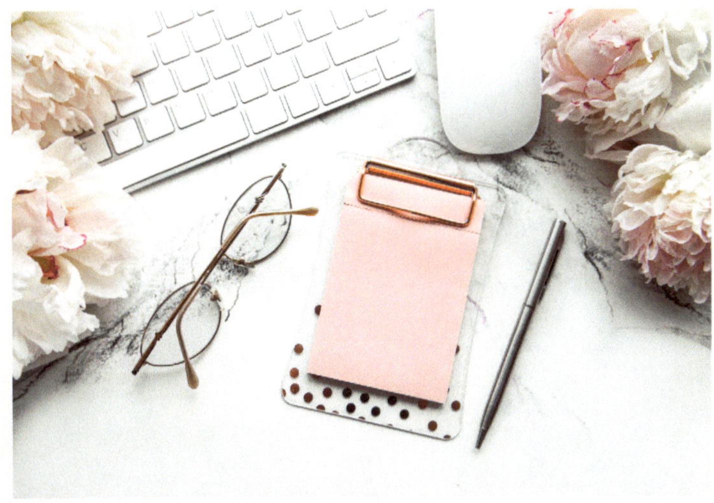

HIV

Human immunodeficiency virus results in Acquired Immunodeficiency Syndrome (AIDS) by killing the key cells of the human immune system known as CD4 cells. This renders the patient unable to fight against many diseases.

HIV in pregnancy is worrisome because it can pass on to the fetus through various means, including:

- HIV can pass to the fetus through the placenta.
- It can pass to the fetus during delivery by exposure to the mother's blood or other fluid.
- Breastfeeding can result in the transmission of HIV from mother to fetus.

Patients with HIV infection are recommended to discuss with their OB steps to be followed to prevent the transmission of the infection to the fetus. Some necessary steps are:

- Using antiviral therapy during pregnancy.
- Using antiviral therapy during labor and delivery.
- Giving birth through cesarean section.
- Do not breastfeed.

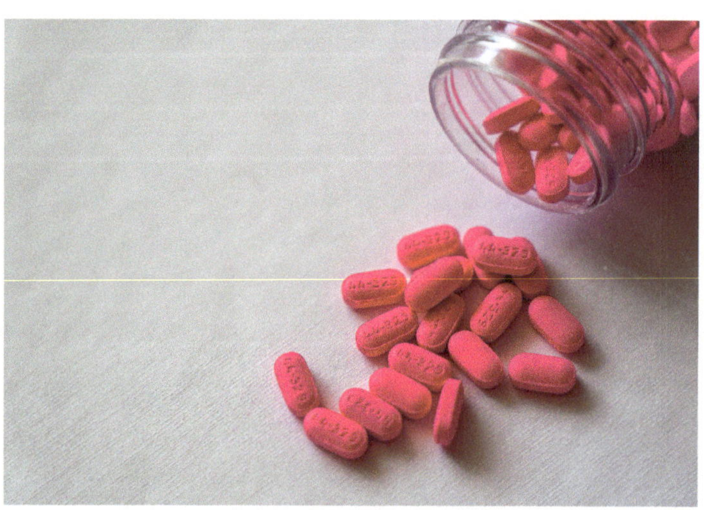

GENITAL HERPES

Genital herpes is a sexually transmitted disease, caused by Human Simplex Virus (HSV) infection. Genital herpes has a risk of transmission from the mother to the fetus during the delivery. The fetus usually gets exposed only while passing through the vaginal canal.

A pregnant woman with an HSV infection should take antiviral medications to shorten the outbreak immediately. Medication is also started at 36 weeks to reduce the chance of an outbreak during delivery. Furthermore, a cesarean section will be preferred as a mode of delivery if an outbreak is present at the time of labor.

UTERINE FIBROIDS

Small fibroids in the wall of the uterus usually display no symptoms and do not affect conception or pregnancy. However, if the fibroid is large or is located within the cavity of the uterus, it can increase your chances of having trouble conceiving, miscarriage, preterm labor, or premature rupture of membranes (breaking the bag of water before labor and before the baby is term). It can sometimes cause placental abruption (detachment of the placenta from the wall of the uterus) and postpartum bleeding. Therefore, patients who have fibroids that meet certain criteria should consider treating the fibroid with an experienced gynecologist before getting pregnant.

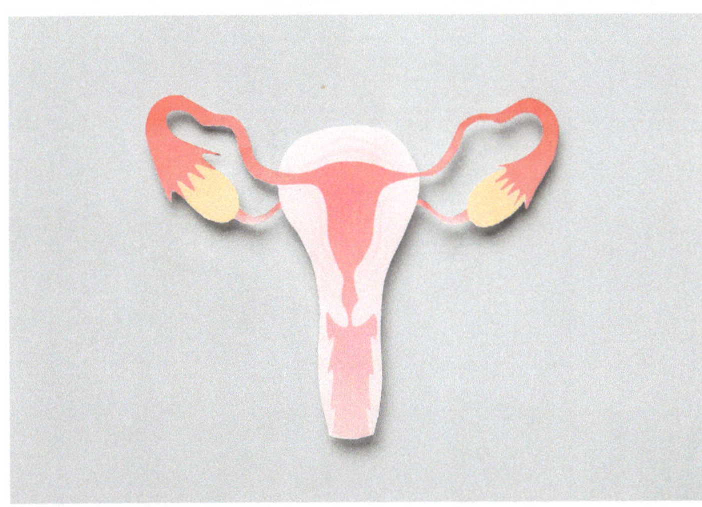

Tips for patients with fibroids

- Management of a patient with fibroids and planning for pregnancy depends on the numbers and size of the fibroids.
- If there are one or more fibroids in the wall of the uterus (not in the cavity) and they are relatively small fibroids (<4cm) that cause no symptoms to the patient, then typically, she can conceive and have a pregnancy without treating the fibroid. All fibroids can, however, cause pain during pregnancy, requiring management.

- If fibroids cause symptoms such as irregular bleeding or pain, then you should discuss with your obstetrician to make a joint decision on whether treating them is the next best course of action before conception.

- When having this discussion with your doctor, make sure you understand the (1) location of each fibroid (2) size, and the implications for conception and pregnancy. Fibroids can be sub-serosal (under the skin of the uterus), intramural (in the wall of the uterine muscle), sub-mucosal (in the cavity), pedunculated (hanging off the uterus via a stem), cervical (sitting in the cervix rather than the uterus) and each represents a different set of possible symptoms and concerns.

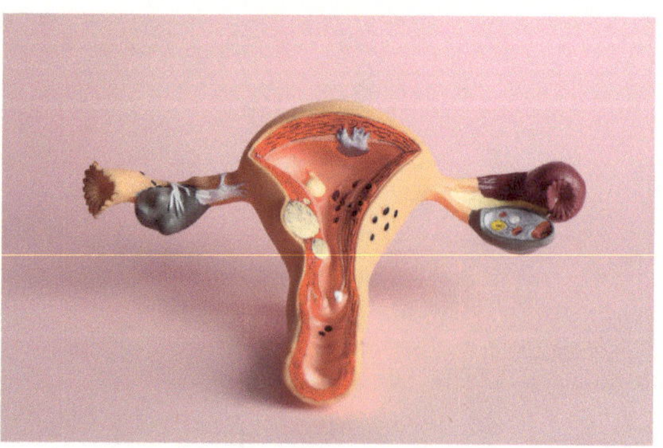

Tips for patients with endometriosis

- Endometriosis is the presence of endometrial tissue outside the uterus. The most common sites are the fallopian tubes, ovaries, and peritoneum. Endometriosis is usually associated with infertility because the inflammation from endometriosis can damage sperm and ovum or interfere with the passage of both sperm and ovum. Severe inflammation sometimes blocks the fallopian tubes causing infertility. (ACOG)
- Some with endometriosis can get pregnant without treatment and it is difficult to predict based on the number or severity of endometriotic lesions. If you have a history of endometriosis, it is important to talk to your doctor if you have not been successful in conceiving after 6-12 months of trying.
- Some anti-inflammatory modalities can be employed to help alleviate symptoms, including taking 1000 mg of ginger rhizome daily, 750 mg of vitamin C daily and turmeric. Although no studies are confirming that this improves pregnancy outcomes, patients report improvement in symptoms.

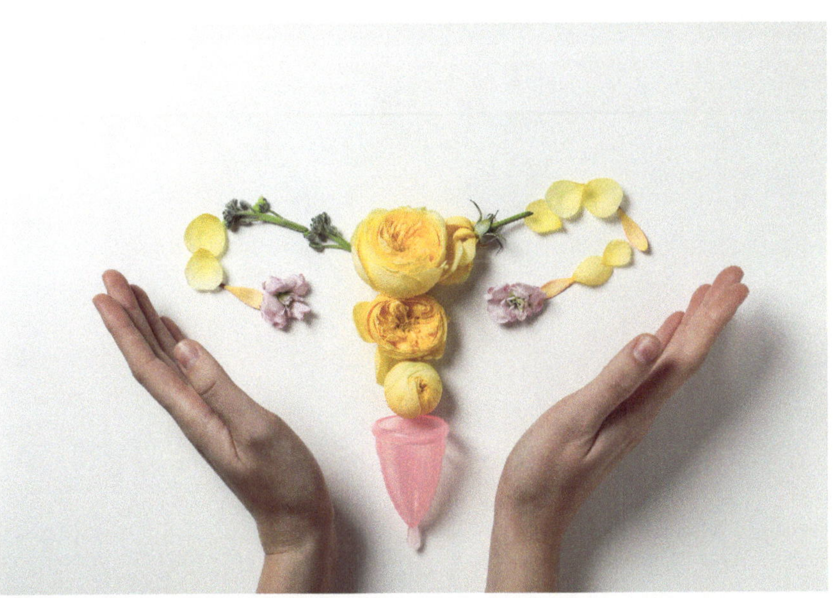

Tips for patients with PCOS (Polycystic ovarian syndrome)

- Polycystic Ovary Syndrome is one of the most common causes of infertility. The main reason for infertility with PCOS is the imbalance of female reproductive hormones that affects the maturation and release of the egg, causing a lack of ovulation. According to ACOG guidelines, the following approaches can increase the chances of pregnancy in a patient with PCOS. (ACOG)
- Obesity is usually associated with PCOS. Weight loss and maintenance of normal weight can help improve the process of ovulation.
- Medications to induce ovulation can be helpful in patients with PCOS. Letrozole, and not clomid*, is now the gold standard for ovulation induction in patients diagnosed with PCOS. Make sure you review effective supplements with your doctor to manage your PCOS as this can naturally help with your fertility.
- If other treatments are not working, surgery of ovaries has also been used, although this is no longer a common practice.
- Assisted reproductive technologies, such as IVF, are also an effective option for patients with PCOS.

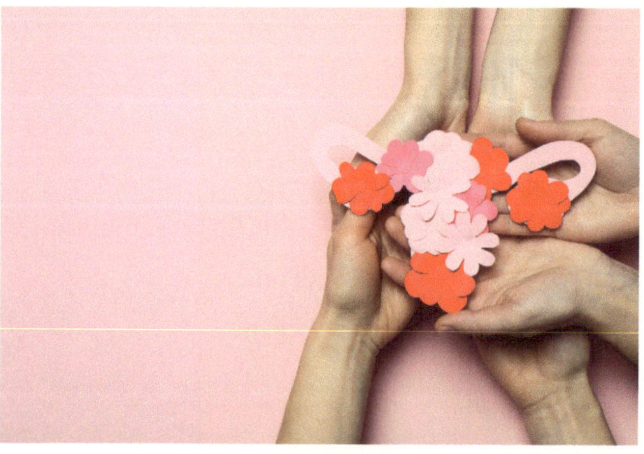

CHAPTER 02

MEDICATIONS TO STOP WHILE TRYING TO CONCEIVE

It is important to know what medications to stop taking when trying to conceive. This chapter will discuss the types of medications to stop while trying to conceive, the reasons why, and the risks associated with continuing to take them. It will also provide advice on how to safely stop taking medications and provide information on the benefits of taking certain medications while trying to conceive.

Types of Medications to Stop While Trying to Conceive

When trying to conceive, it is important to stop taking certain medications to avoid unnecessary exposure to the fetus. By the time you get a positive pregnancy test result, your baby has already begun developing vital organs. The types of medications that should be stopped include:

1. **Hormonal birth control**: This one is pretty obvious however it comes up often enough as a question that I decided to include it here. Hormonal birth control, such as the pill, patch, and ring, should be stopped when trying to conceive. These medications contain hormones that interfere with ovulation, making it difficult to conceive.

2. **Certain antibiotics**: Certain antibiotics, such as tetracycline, minocycline, and doxycycline, can interfere with the development of a fetus and should be stopped when trying to conceive.

3. **Nonsteroidal anti-inflammatory drugs (NSAIDs)**: NSAIDs, such as ibuprofen and naproxen, can increase the risk of miscarriage and other cardiac problems in the fetus once pregnant. They should be avoided whenever possible.

4. **Certain antidepressants**: Certain antidepressants, such as selective serotonin reuptake inhibitors (SSRIs), can increase the risk of miscarriage however carefully evaluate the specific medication, and discuss the risks/benefits of staying on it with your psychiatrist.

5. **Certain anxiety medications**: Certain anxiety medications, such as benzodiazepines should be avoided

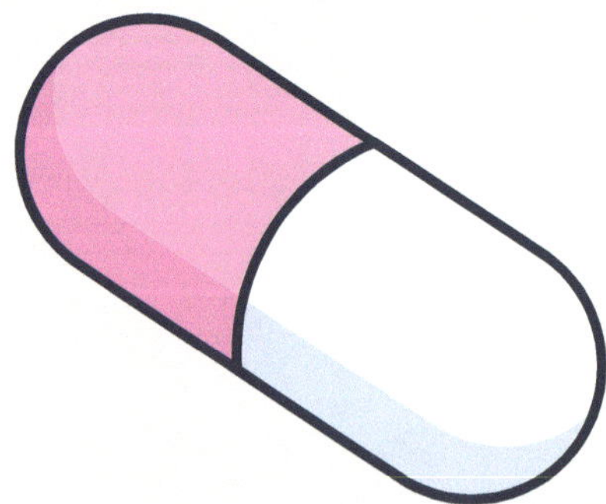

Although the list is too long to include in this book in its entirety, some common ones that I see often in patients who present for preconception counseling are mentioned below. Your medications should be carefully evaluated by your obstetrician during a preconception counseling visit. You should never stop any medication without the guidance of your prescribing physician and OBGYN.

- Methotrexate.
- ACE inhibitors. These are used to treat hypertension.
- Tetracycline (antibiotic)
- Valproic acid. It is used to treat epileptic conditions
- Isotretinoin. It is used to treat acne.
- NSAIDs such as Ibuprofen and naproxen (Common American brands are ALEVE, ADVIL, and PAMPRIN) are also not recommended in pregnancy. These can be used before conception, however.
- Certain anti-epileptic drugs
- Antipsychotics like risperidone
- Spironolactone has anti-androgenic activities and can affect the developing male fetus
- Warfarin
- Ribavirin
- Triazolam
- Aliskiren
- Bosentan
- Methylene blue
- Oxytocin
- Levonorgestrel
- Isotretinoin
- Griseofulvin
- Riociguat

Again, If you are on a medication that is not safe in pregnancy, do not stop them abruptly without speaking with your doctor. You may need to find a reasonable alternative to manage your current condition safely.

CHAPTER 03

One of the key components of a healthy pregnancy is maintaining a healthy weight before conception. This chapter will provide an overview of the importance of weight management before pregnancy and discuss the potential risks associated with obesity and being underweight during pregnancy. It will also provide information on how to manage weight with diet and exercise before becoming pregnant.

The Importance of Weight Management Before Pregnancy

Women need to be at a healthy weight when they become pregnant. Women who are overweight or obese before becoming pregnant may be at higher risk for complications during pregnancy and childbirth. Several studies have found that obese women are more likely to have longer labor, cesarean sections, and postpartum infections. In addition, obese women are more likely to develop gestational diabetes and high blood pressure. Furthermore, studies have found that obese women are more likely to have larger babies, and babies born to obese women are more likely to be born prematurely. Being overweight can increase your chances of miscarriage, fetal death, pregnancy complications such as hypertension, pre-eclampsia, gestational diabetes, abnormal fetal growth and increase your risk for a cesarian section. If a caesarian section is performed, obesity puts you at risk for poor wound healing, blood clots, hemorrhage, and more.

WEIGHT MANAGEMENT

Losing just 5% of your current body weight can increase your chance of healthier pregnancy outcomes by several folds. Set yourself a realistic goal and get help from either your OBGYN, a nutritionist, or your primary care provider so that you can reach a healthier weight. If you are under the age of 35, giving yourself 3-6 months to attain a healthier weight can make a big difference in your journey.

On the other hand, underweight women may also be at risk for complications during pregnancy and childbirth. Studies have found that underweight women are more likely to have smaller babies and to have a higher risk of premature delivery. In addition, underweight women are more likely to have a higher risk of postpartum depression. Being underweight can also lead to difficulty getting pregnant, miscarriage, and fetal growth problems.

Planning for pregnancy puts you in the ideal place of being able to achieve a healthy weight if your BMI is abnormal before you conceive, improving your chances for better outcomes.
The ranges of BMI are:

Underweight = 18.5 or lower
Healthy weight = 18.5 to 24.9
Overweight = 25 to 29.9
Obesity = 30 and above

WEIGHT MANAGEMENT

You can use easy online calculators to enter your height and weight and obtain your BMI. Remember that BMI does not tell the entire story. For example, central obesity, where a woman carries most of her weight in her abdomen, will pose a greater risk for poor cesarian section outcome than someone with a similar BMI but has a better hip-to-waist ratio where most of their fat is not carried centrally.

 **Effect of low BMI on Pregnancy**

An underweight mother is at risk of giving birth to a low-birth-weight child. Low birth weight babies can face complications during labor and after birth. The risk of preterm birth also increases with low BMI.

If your BMI is less than 18.5, you need to eat high-caloric food daily to improve your weight to the normal level of BMI. Prenatal vitamins are also recommended to avoid any nutritional deficiency.

Effect of high BMI on Pregnancy:

A list of well-known risks include:

- Hypertension
- Pre-eclampsia
- Preterm birth
- Gestational diabetes
- Neural tubes defects
- Macrosomic baby
- Birth injuries
- Increased risk of requiring a C-section
- Wound healing problems

CHAPTER 04
MENTAL HEALTH

Nearly 1 in 5 women in the United States currently have a diagnosis of anxiety, depression, bipolar disease, ADHD, or other mental health diagnoses. A woman's mental health before pregnancy is a critical issue for both expectant mothers and their unborn children. Pre-pregnancy mental health can have profound implications for the health and development of a fetus. Therefore, it is important for women to be aware of potential risks and to take steps to improve their mental health before conceiving. This chapter will provide an overview of the current literature on pre-pregnancy mental health, including the risks associated with poor mental health before pregnancy, as well as strategies for managing mental health before pregnancy.

There is a growing body of research that suggests that mental health before pregnancy can have a significant impact on the health of the unborn child. Studies have found that women who experience depression or anxiety before pregnancy are more likely to experience complications during pregnancy, such as preterm labor or low birth weight. Additionally, there is evidence that pre-pregnancy mental health can have an impact on the long-term health of the child, including increased risk of developmental delays and behavioral problems.

MENTAL HEALTH

Furthermore, pre-pregnancy mental health has been linked to an increased risk of substance abuse during pregnancy. Women who are dealing with mental health issues before pregnancy may be more likely to turn to alcohol or drugs as a coping mechanism during pregnancy. This can have serious consequences for the fetus, including fetal alcohol syndrome, birth defects, and other health complications.

Women with a mental health diagnosis are at increased risk of developing postpartum depression or psychosis, two conditions that can be very dangerous to the mother and newborn's well-being. Avoid conception if you feel that your treatment is not yet optimized.

You will need to work very closely with your psychiatrist and therapist, letting them know of your plans to conceive so that they can devise a medical treatment plan to stabilize your symptoms and get you ready for a safe pregnancy. It is important not to suddenly discontinue your medications before speaking with your providers as some medications carry severe withdrawal symptoms or can cause your mental health to spiral.

MENTAL HEALTH

Women need to take steps to reduce stress and improve their overall well-being before pregnancy. This can include engaging in regular physical activity, practicing relaxation techniques, and engaging in activities that bring joy and happiness. Additionally, it can be helpful to create a support network of family and friends that can provide emotional support.

Finally, women need to practice healthy eating habits. Malnutrition or deficiencies of essential nutrients can have an impact on mental health and can be especially detrimental during pregnancy. Therefore, it is important to eat a balanced diet and to take prenatal vitamins to ensure that the need for all essential nutrients are being met.

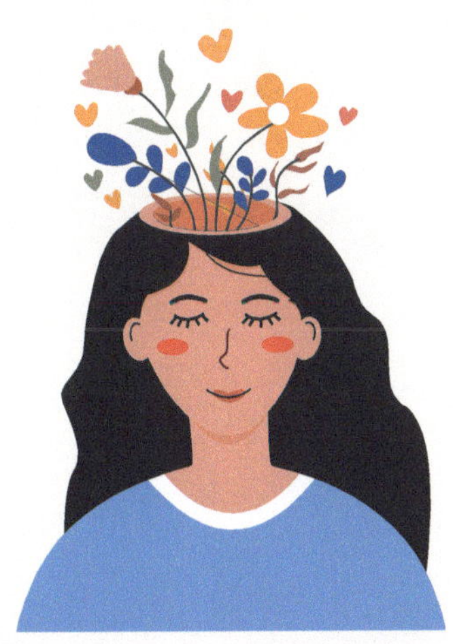

MENTAL HEALTH

Below are some common psychiatric medications that are generally safe:

- Clozapine
- Benztropine
- Methylphenidate
- Buspirone
- Zolpidem
- Maprotiline
- Bupropion

Below are some common psychiatric medications to discuss with your doctors.

- Diazepam
- Alprazolam
- Midazolam
- Lithium
- Topiramate
- Phenytoin
- Carbamazepine
- Flurazepam
- Triazolam
- Paroxetine

CHAPTER 05

NUTRITION AND SUPPLEMENTS

A healthy diet is the key to good physical health. A healthy diet contains essential nutrients. Here are a few general tips to achieve this:

- A woman should consume more whole foods, fruits, and vegetables containing essential minerals and vitamins.
- Protein-containing foods such as meat, fish, chicken, and dairy products are also recommended.
- Processed foods should generally be avoided.
- Smoking and alcohol consumption should also be avoided because they can cause complications during pregnancy.

Before pregnancy, a Mediterranean or low carbohydrate diet is the most conducive to conception.

Once pregnancy occurs, there will be certain foods to avoid.

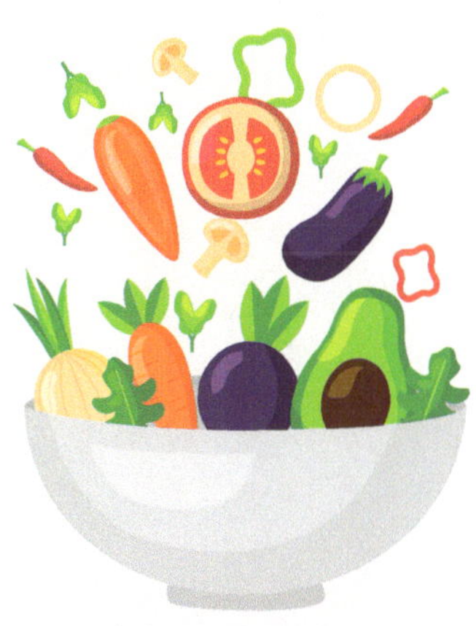

Pregnant women should avoid certain types of foods that can increase their risk of developing foodborne illnesses. These foods include raw, undercooked, or contaminated meats, poultry, and seafood; unpasteurized milk and dairy products; and raw eggs. Additionally, pregnant women should avoid processed deli meats, soft cheeses, and foods made with raw eggs, such as mayonnaise and certain types of dressings.

Caffeine

Large volumes of caffeinated beverages, such as coffee, tea, and soda, should be avoided during pregnancy. High levels of caffeine can cause dehydration and increase the risk of miscarriage although this data isn't clear. The American College of Obstetricians and Gynecologists recommends limiting caffeine intake to less than 200 mg per day.

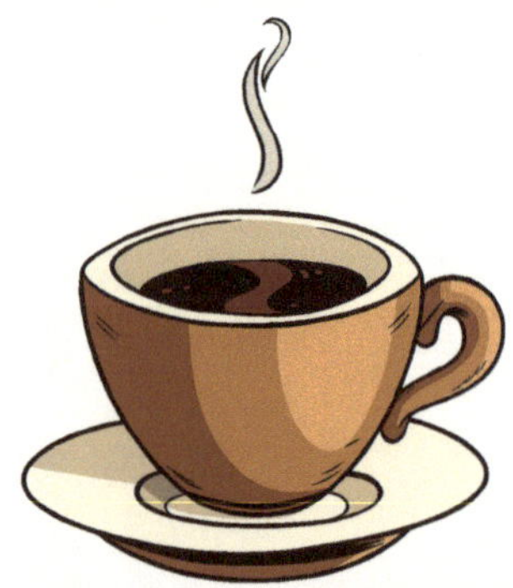

Alcohol should be avoided completely during pregnancy. Drinking alcohol during pregnancy can cause fetal alcohol syndrome, which can lead to physical and mental disabilities in the unborn baby.

Fish High in Mercury

Fish that are high in mercury, such as swordfish, shark, tilefish, and king mackerel, should be avoided during pregnancy. Mercury can be toxic to a developing fetus and can cause developmental delays and other health problems.

Unwashed Fruits and Vegetables

Pregnant women should make sure to wash all fruits and vegetables before eating them, as unwashed produce can contain harmful bacteria and parasites.

Herbs and Supplements

Pregnant women should also be cautious with non-culinary herbal supplements, as some of these may contain ingredients that are unsafe for the fetus or can even trigger uterine contractions. It is best to check with a doctor or pharmacist before taking any during pregnancy.

Supplements:

During pregnancy, the demand for certain elements is increased by the body and this demand is often not met by the standard American diet. Therefore, proper intake of the necessary nutrients is important to avoid complications during pregnancy.

Some of the important supplements recommended before pregnancy are given below.

- **Vitamins**: Vitamins play a key role in maintaining the body's functions. Therefore, one serving per day of prenatal vitamins is recommended.
- **Calcium**: Calcium is well known for its role in the formation and strengthening of the bones and teeth of the newborn.
- **Folic Acid:** Folic Acid is important for preventing mother anemia and the newborn's neural tube defects. A daily dose of 400 micrograms per day is recommended by ACOG however if you were diagnosed with PCOS or infertility, increase this to a minimum of 800 mcg a day.

- **Iron**: Iron is an essential element of red blood cells and its need increases in pregnancy. Therefore, adequate supplementation of iron is necessary. Women should take prenatal vitamins with iron or consume iron-rich foods such as cereals, beans, liver, and beef.

The easiest way to ensure that you are getting what you need is to start an approved prenatal vitamin 6 months before you conceive and then stay on this through 12 weeks after having your baby or when you complete breastfeeding. As a bonus, they are partially responsible for your pregnancy glow as well!

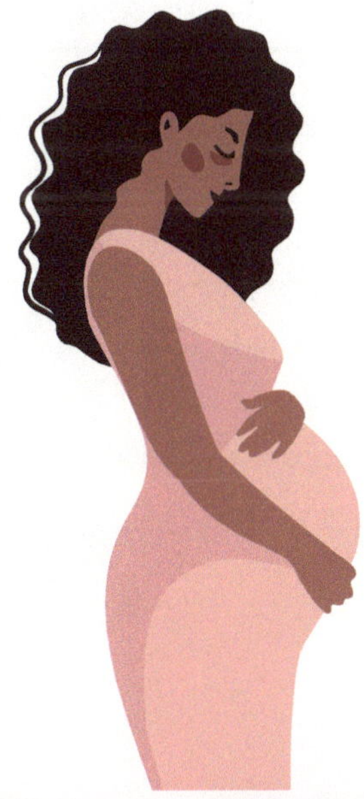

CHAPTER 06

SHOULD I CHECK ON MY FERTILITY?

According to ACOG <u>recommendations</u>, you need to check on your fertility if you are unsuccessful in getting pregnant for one year despite regular sexual intercourse without any birth control. Women aged 35 and above should evaluate their fertility after trying conception for 6 months.

Are you having a monthly, relatively pain-free period/cycle?

Regular periods indicate normal ovulation. If you are skipping periods or have varying lengths between one period to another, it may point to hormonal disorders, such as PCOS, that will need to be evaluated. Heavy pain during menstruation may point to certain conditions such as endometriosis or adenomyosis, fibroids, ovarian cysts, or infections that may alter your conception discussion.

Do you have a history of recurrent miscarriages?

Talk to your OBGYN about the details of your history to determine if further investigation is warranted

SHOULD I CHECK ON MY FERTILITY?

Do you have a strong family history of infertility and have been trying for 6 months without success?

Although this does not meet the official criteria for testing, consider having a personalized discussion with your OBGYN to see if testing can be started sooner based on your clinical history, even if you are younger than 35.

Do you have a history of fibroids, cysts, polyps, or other gynecological problems?

If you have a history of fibroids or other gynecological pathologies such as cysts, polyps, etc, discuss a pelvic ultrasound and any other necessary testing with your OBGYN.

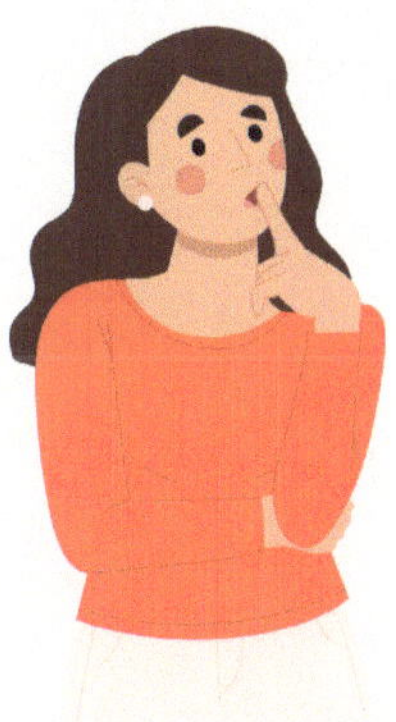

TESTS YOU CAN PERFORM AT HOME:

There are simple tests that can be performed at home to assess for monthly ovulation:

Monitoring of basal body temperature (BBT):

The basal body temperature of women rises around ovulation for 2-3 days. You can record your ovulation days by noting your body temperature in the morning for 2-3 cycles and observing for patterns. Before ovulation, your BBT may range from about 97.2 to 97.7 degrees F. But the day after you ovulate, you should see an uptick of 0.5 to 1.0 degrees in your BBT, which should last until about your next period. Please note that there are certain conditions and environmental reasons which may not allow you to notice this difference so don't solely rely on your BBT.

Cervical mucus monitoring:

A woman can identify her ovulation days and fertile period by regularly monitoring her cervical mucus. Cervical mucus becomes thin, stretchy, and slippery (like an egg white) just before ovulation.

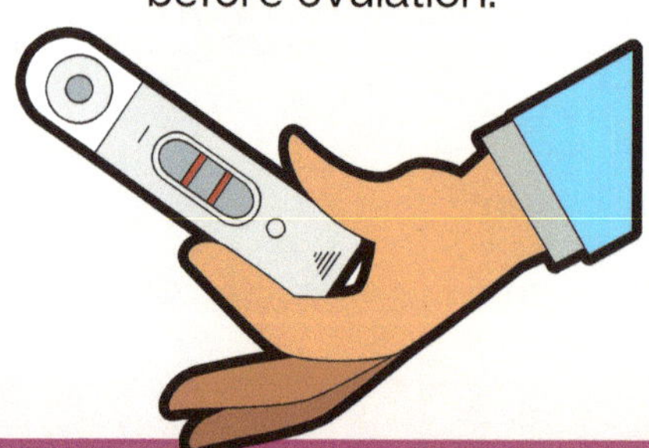

Ovulation Test Strips:

Ovulation test strips are another good option to evaluate your fertility days and ovulation at home. Strips measure the levels of Luteinizing hormone in the urine to predict ovulation. While performing the test, the following steps should be followed:

- Beginning the day after your menstrual cycle ends, catch a urine sample in a clean cup. Place the absorbing end of the strip in the urine for at least 10 seconds.
- Wait for no more than 5 minutes and then read your strip.
- Two lines should always appear: A dark control line which is furthest away from the absorbing end, and your result line. If only 1 line appears, discard and use a new strip.
- If the test line appears dark or darker than the control line, your test is positive and you are going to ovulate within the next 12-36 hours.
- If the test line appears lighter than the control line, your test is negative. You have to repeat the test daily at the same time until you get a positive result.
- If you never get a positive result, you may have either missed the ovulation, or you did not ovulate and you should discuss this further with your OBGYN.

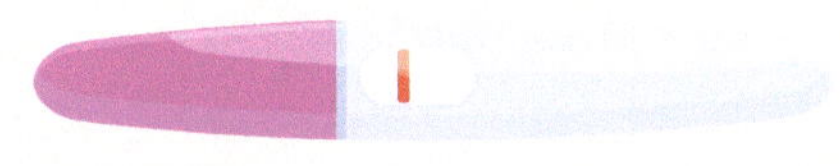

When is the best time to have intercourse?

Timed intercourse is key for a successful conception. It is important to remember that you want the sperm ready and present by the time the egg has been released. This means that the best time to have intercourse is about 2 days before the positive ovulation test, the day of the positive test, and the 2 days following the positive test. A positive test simply means that the LH surge has been detected. This in turn means that the egg will be released in the next 36 hours so don't miss the 2 days following a positive ovulation test. Although healthy sperm can live for up to 5 days, the ejaculated sperm will have varying life spans.

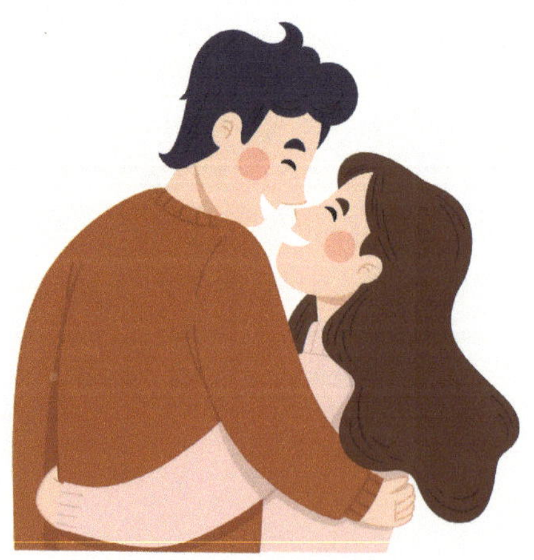

TESTS ORDERED BY YOUR DOCTOR

Labs

FSH TEST:

- FSH test reveals the levels of follicle-stimulating hormone in the blood. Follicle Stimulating Hormone (FSH) is released by the pituitary gland and it controls the formation of eggs in the ovaries as well as regulates the menstrual cycle.

- Ideal values will be below 20. During a cycle, FSH reaches its peak at the time of ovulation.

AMH TEST:

- AMH is the level of anti-Mullerian hormone in the serum. AMH is released by the eggs present in the ovaries therefore, AMH levels can reflect the egg reserve.
- The ideal value of AMH in serum is between 1 and 3 however normal goes up to 6.8 ng/ml. Normal levels of AMH indicate an adequate amount of eggs that can be fertilized for conception. However, very low levels of AMH signify a deficient amount of fertilizable eggs. Values less than 1 can suggest peri-menopause and should be discussed with your doctor. Values above 7 may suggest problems with ovulation and should also be discussed.

LH, Testosterone, DHEA-S, Prolactin, estradiol, TSH/T4:
This full hormonal panel can help diagnose other issues that can make it difficult to conceive and will be ordered at the same time as your FSH and AMH test.

Pelvic ultrasound
If you have a history of fibroids or other gynecological pathologies such as cysts, polyps, painful periods, pelvic pain, irregular cycles and more request a pelvic ultrasound. A pelvic ultrasound will display the current status of the uterus, fallopian tubes, and ovaries and will identify the abnormal conditions that can interfere with fertility such as fibroids, cysts, or polyps if present. Changes in the follicles inside the ovaries can also be observed through ultrasound.

Sonohysterography is another ultrasound technique that is used to examine pathologies inside the uterus if the ultrasound suggests an abnormality within the cavity such as a possible fibroid in the cavity or a polyp.

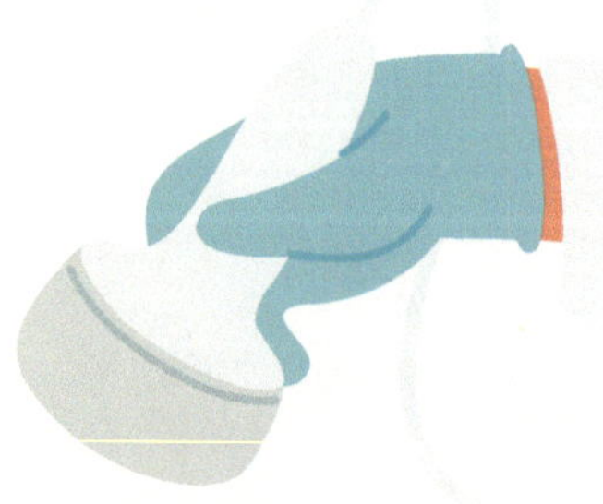

HSG(Hysterosalpingogram) and Semen analysis

If you have been trying for 6-12 months without success, it may be time to check and see whether or not you have any blockage in the tubes. This can be caused by prior infections, fluid in the tube and even scarring from old surgeries (such as a cesarian section to name one). A dye is injected into the uterus at a radiology center under an X-ray machine and pictures are taken to make sure that the dye fills the cavity and spills out of both tubes in real time.

It is also important to remember that 40% of infertility cases are male in origin, so have your partner get an order for a semen analysis as well.

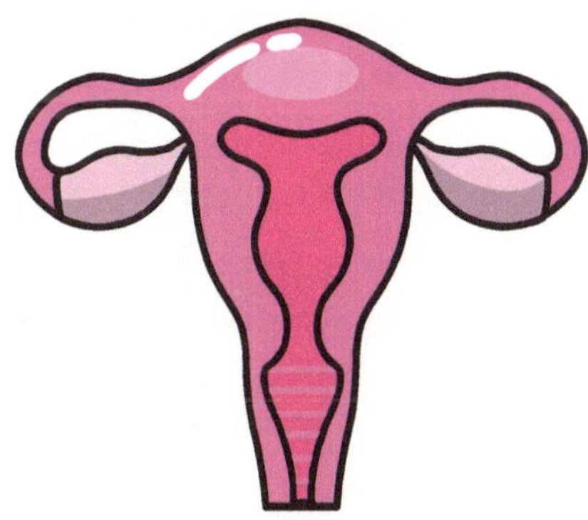

Additional tests and procedures that may come up in your conversation:

- **Hysteroscopy:** In this technique, a camera with a light source is used to examine the interior of the uterus and can also guide minor surgical procedures. This is helpful if your ultrasound shows a pathology in the cavity that needs to be confirmed or sampled. Many OBGYNs offer this quickly and safely in the office.

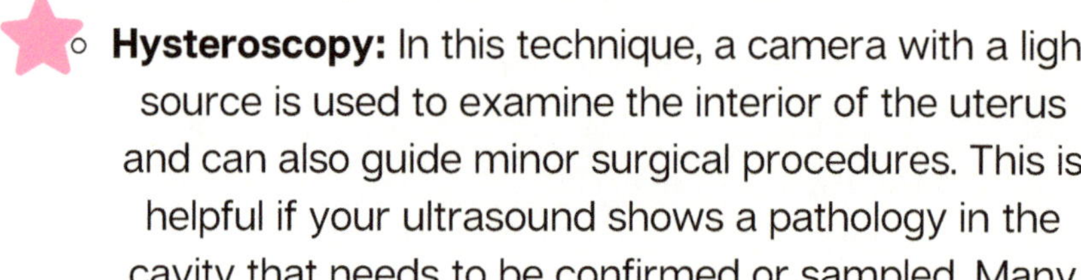

- **Sonohysterography:** A special ultrasound technique where the technician takes pictures while your doctor slowly injects sterile saline in the uterine cavity. This is useful is diagnosing any pathology in the endometrium of the uterus (inner cavity).

- **Laparoscopy:** It is a diagnostic as well as a therapeutic technique in which a camera with a light source is inserted through the abdomen to see the uterus, fallopian tubes, and ovaries. This is done under general anesthesia in a hospital and is only reserved for severe cases of infertility where endometriosis is suspected.

CHAPTER 07

Sperm health and conception is an essential topic for couples looking to conceive a child. With advances in medical technology, couples are now able to increase their chances of conception by understanding the importance of sperm health, and how to improve it. The purpose of this chapter is to provide an overview of sperm health and conception and to discuss the various factors that can affect fertility.

Sperm Health and Fertility

Sperm health is essential for successful conception. Sperm health is affected by a variety of factors including environmental, lifestyle, and genetic factors. The quality and quantity of sperm are important factors in successful conception. Poor sperm health can result in lower sperm counts and lower motility, which can result in decreased fertility.

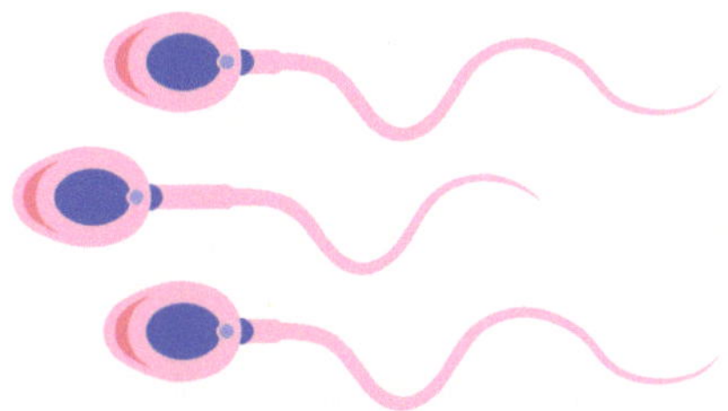

Environmental Factors

Environmental factors can have a significant impact on sperm health and fertility. Exposure to environmental toxins, such as cigarette smoke, air pollutants, and radiation, can affect sperm health. Additionally, exposure to certain chemicals, such as pesticides, can also affect sperm health. It is also important to note that certain medications, such as antibiotics and anti-inflammatory drugs, can also affect it.

Lifestyle Factors

Lifestyle habits can also have a significant impact on sperm health and fertility. Excessive alcohol consumption, smoking, and drug use can all affect sperm health.

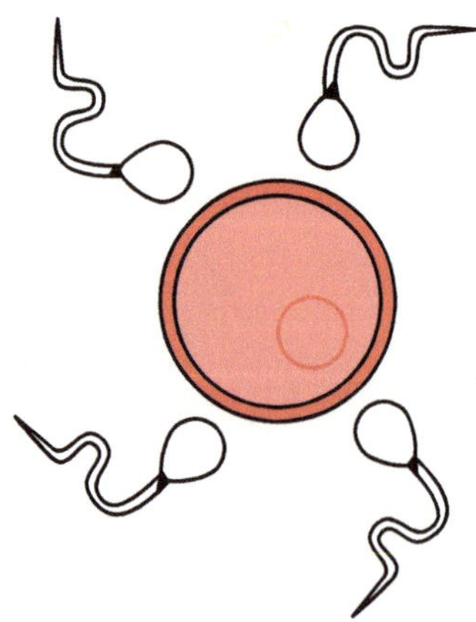

Genetic Factors

Genetic factors can play a role in sperm health and fertility. Certain genetic diseases, such as cystic fibrosis, can cause reduced fertility or infertility. Additionally, certain inherited conditions, such as sickle cell anemia, can also affect sperm.

Role of Medical Science

Medical science has made great strides in improving sperm health and fertility. Various treatments, such as hormone therapy, can be used to improve sperm health. In addition to medical treatments, lifestyle modifications, such as diet and exercise, can also help improve sperm health. Have your partner see a urologist if the semen analysis is showing some significant abnormalities.

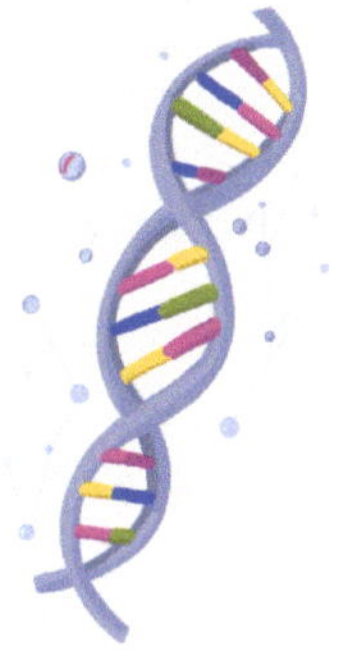

Tips for partner's sperm health

Occasionally a problem with men's reproductive system turns out to be the cause of infertility. The following are some tests that can be used to assess the reproductive functions of a male partner:

- **Semen Analysis:** This test demonstrates the amount of sperm (sperm count) in males, the shape and size of the sperm, as well as its motility. It is a useful tool to assess the sperm health of a male partner.
- **Testosterone Levels:** Testosterone is a male reproductive hormone that controls sperm production and sexual function. Altered levels of testosterone can interfere with normal sperm count and sexual function.
- **Ultrasound**: A scrotum ultrasound can be performed to see any pathology in the testicles if the semen analysis is abnormal.

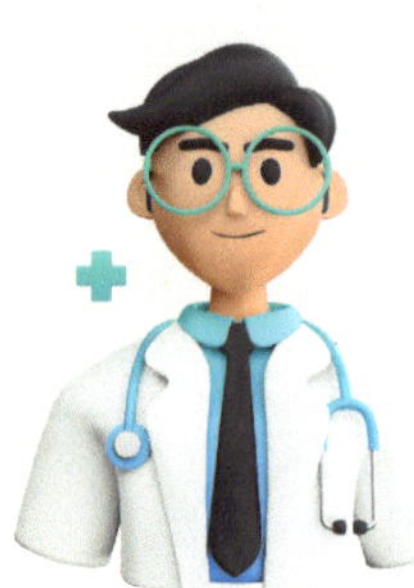

SPERM HEALTH

What can men do to keep their sperm healthy?

The following are some lifestyle modifications that can boost your partner's sperm health as well as sperm count:

- Quit smoking
- Quit Alcohol
- Maintain your weight within the normal BMI range
- Avoid tight clothes around the testes
- Avoid jacuzzis
- Avoid hot showers, hot baths
- Eat fresh fruits and vegetables
- Drink 2L of water a day
- Limit caffeine consumption
- Exercise regularly
- Take fertility vitamins for men
- Eat a balanced diet
-

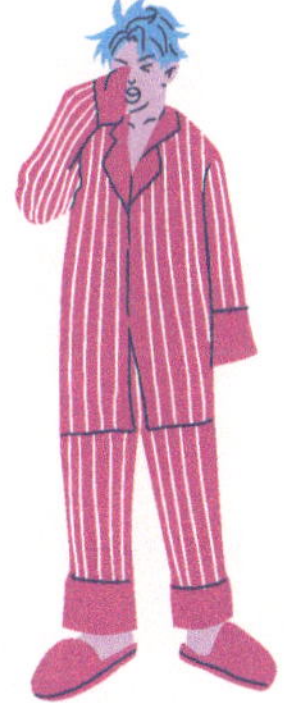

CHAPTER 08

Quitting the current birth control and regaining fertility depends on the type of birth control method. Various birth control methods are discussed below:

The combination pill, patch, and ring
The combination pills, also known as combined oral contraceptives, vaginal rings, and skin patches prevent pregnancy by releasing estrogen and progestin hormones. Both these hormones prevent the ovulation process resulting in birth control.

You can return to your baseline fertility within 4 weeks of stopping the combination pills or removing your skin patch or vaginal ring. However, it may take a female up to 3 months to get back to her regular cycle after stopping the pills. Make sure to talk to your OBGYN if this occurs while trying to conceive.

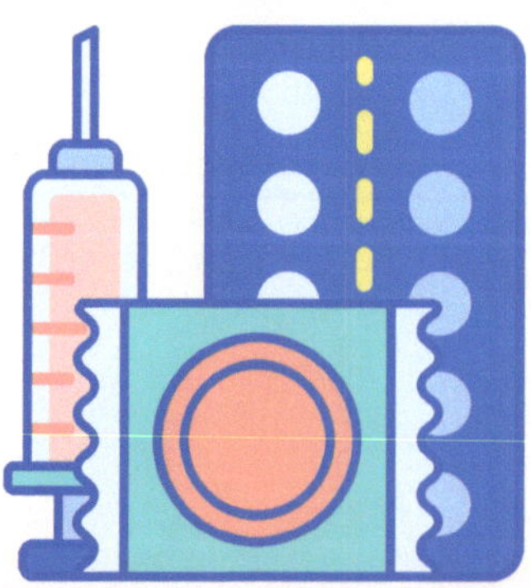

The progesterone-only pill

The progesterone-only pills contain the progestin hormone which inhibits pregnancy by stopping ovulation and thickening the cervical mucus.

According to the ACOG guidelines, return to baseline fertility is more rapid than seen with combination pills.

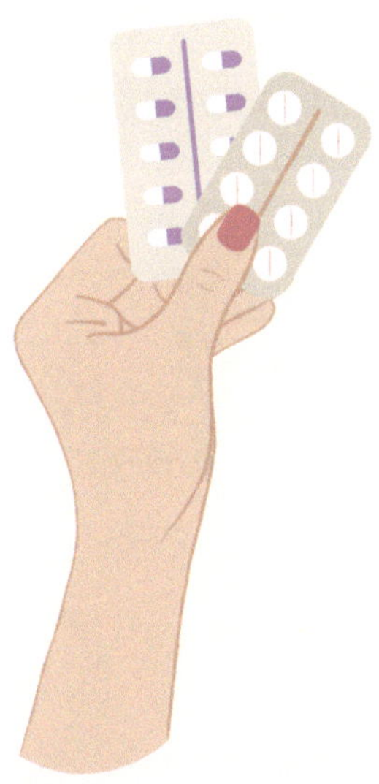

The IUD (intra-uterine device)

The intrauterine device is a small usually T-shaped device that is placed in the uterus to prevent pregnancy. Intrauterine devices are of two types: one is hormonal which releases the progestin hormone and the other is Copper-containing which releases copper ions to stop the fusion of sperm and ovum.

If you are planning a pregnancy, just have your OBGYN remove your IUD and you can expect to return to baseline fertility within your next menstrual cycle which can take up to 4-6 weeks after removal.

The Depo shot

The Depo shot is a progesterone injection that contains the medroxyprogesterone hormone and provides contraception for 3 months by inhibiting ovulation and thickening the cervical mucus.

ACOG guidelines state that it may take an average of 10 months to get back to baseline fertility after quitting the injection. In some females, it may take 1-2 years to regain normal fertility after stopping the Depo shot.

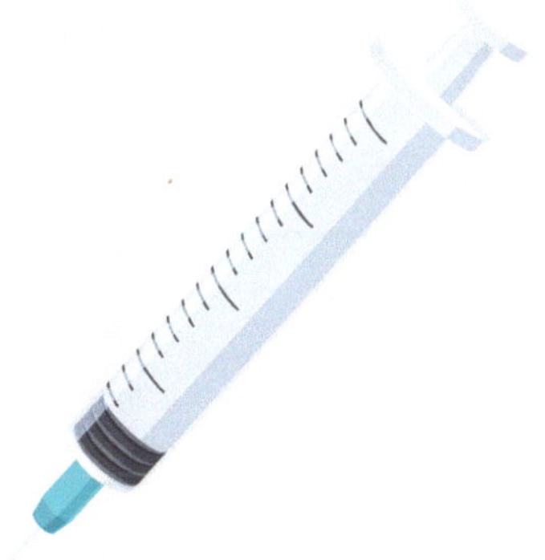

The progesterone implant

The progesterone implant is a small rod about the size of a matchstick. It is inserted in the upper arm below the skin. The implant releases the progesterone hormone and prevents pregnancy by interfering with ovulation.

Generally, your baseline fertility returns as soon as the next cycle after removing the implant.

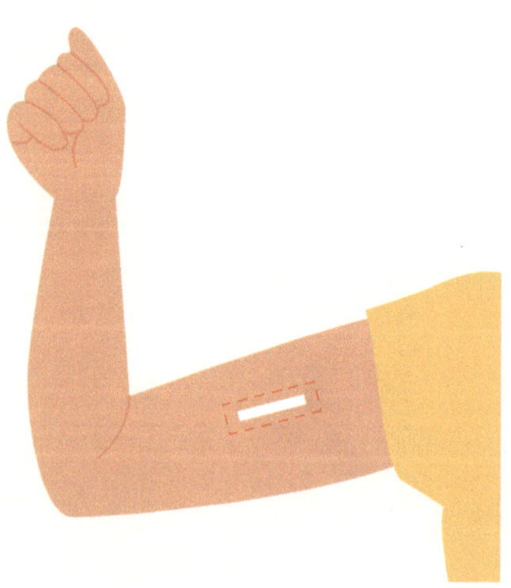

Did you have a tubal ligation or sterilization surgery?

Tubal ligation or sterilization is considered a permanent technique of contraception for women. In this technique, fallopian tubes are either removed or closed off by a surgical procedure. This prevents the movement of the egg through the tubes to fuse with the sperm thus causing birth control.

What are my options?

Reversal Options:

Although tubal ligations are considered an irreversible technique there are a few doctors who still offer reversal through surgery. The surgery may have complications and may not guarantee that you will regain fertility. (ACOG)

Another option to get pregnant after tubal ligation is **assisted reproductive technology.**

This technology essentially allows you to bypass the tubes by inserting an already fertilized embryo directly into the uterus via in-vitro fertilization (IVF). In this technique, sperm and egg are combined outside the body, in a laboratory. The embryo is then transferred to the uterus.

CHAPTER 09

A pregnancy and delivery team includes various health professionals who provide you with care and assistance during pregnancy as well as at the time of delivery.
A board-certified obstetrician is the pillar of your pregnancy and delivery team. Other healthcare providers in your team may include a maternal-fetal medicine specialist, a doula, a midwife, a pediatrician, and any specialists you see for specific chronic ongoing conditions.

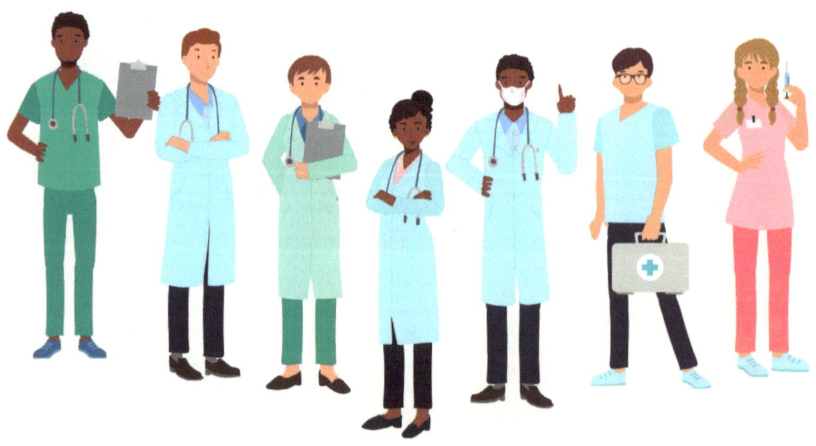

How to choose the right OBGYN

An obstetrician plays a key role in providing care during your pregnancy as well as at your child's birth. Therefore, it is necessary to choose the right OBGYN. You should consider the following aspects while choosing the right OBGYN:

- Choose an OBGYN who is board-certified and experienced or is part of a network of colleagues who meet these criteria.
- Choose an OBGYN with whom you feel relaxed and comfortable.
- Research the delivering hospital location and make sure it is within 30 minutes from your home or less by car.

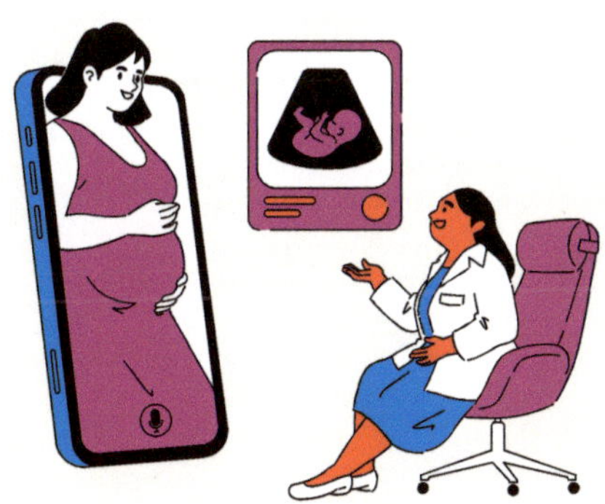

How to choose the right OBGYN (continued)

- Research the NICU level of the delivering hospital and ensure that there is at least a level 2 NICU available, and level 3 if you have any high-risk conditions. This determines what the neonatal center at that hospital can handle should it occur with your baby without having to transfer them out to another hospital. See below for an explanation of the different levels.

- If you are from a minority background, consider choosing an OBGYN from a similar background or one who is known for having robust diversity training. It is important to see a physician who not only understands you but will also not dismiss you or change their practice patterns due to unconscious bias. Compared to white women, black women have a three to four times higher risk of dying from pregnancy-related reasons. Choose a physician who never dismisses your symptoms and acknowledges and respects your experience and perspective.

What in the world is a NICU level?

A hospital with a Level II NICU can care for:

- Stable or moderately ill newborn infants born at or after 32 weeks gestation and who weigh at least 1,500 grams (3.3 pounds)
- Babies who are full-term but who require close monitoring for issues like jaundice or trouble staying warm
- Newborns whose problems are expected to resolve rapidly and are not expected to need sub-specialty level services urgently (like a pediatric heart or breathing specialist).

-

Level II NICU resources and services include:

- Assisted or mechanical ventilation (to help the newborn breathe) on a short-term basis, preferably under 24 hours
- Some specialized equipment, for example, a portable X-ray machine and blood gas analyzer
- Medical staff who are available continuously for ongoing care, in case of emergencies and have special training in neonatal (newborn) care

Babies who cannot breathe on their own 24 hours after birth should be transferred to a higher level of care.

What in the world is a NICU level?

What is a Level III NICU?

Level III (three) NICUs provide critical care for babies born before 32 weeks gestation or babies with specific medical conditions that require surgery or other specialized pediatric care.

A hospital with a Level III NICU is equipped to care for:

- Preterm infants born before 32 weeks or who weigh less than 1,500 grams (3.3 pounds) at birth
- Babies with medical or surgical conditions, regardless of age

A Level III NICU must:

- Have significant clinical experience demonstrated by large patient volumes and complexity of care
- Have neonatal and pediatric subspecialists available promptly, 24/7 (though not necessarily on-site)
- Be able to provide life support for as long as needed
- Have quick access to specialized newborn services including surgery, advanced breathing support, specialized monitoring equipment, nutrition, pharmacy, and imaging services.

What is a Level IV NICU?

Level IV (four) NICUs offer the highest level of medical care for newborns and premature infants with high-risk conditions. These facilities are equipped to care for the most complex neonatal conditions and the sickest and smallest newborns, no matter their gestational age at birth. There are very few across the country and your doctor may recommend one if your baby is diagnosed with a critical condition before birth.

These facilities have all the capabilities of a Level III NICU, plus they employ more experienced staff with 24/7 access to medical and surgical specialists who care only for children. Level IV NICUs provide the same services as Level III NICUs and:

- Continuous, on-site care from pediatric medical and pediatric surgery subspecialists, such as children's heart, brain, and lung specialists
- Surgery for complex conditions present at birth (known as congenital conditions)

The role of the fetal medicine specialist

If you have a medical condition that makes you a high-risk pregnancy, it is important that you see both an MFM (Maternal Fetal Medicine Specialist) as well as your OBGYN. They will work closely together to give you and your baby the best outcome. Most MFMs also offer preconception counseling where you can discuss key aspects of your pregnancy planning and how to optimize your health before conceiving.

The role of the pediatrician

A pediatrician plays a key role at the time of a child's birth, however, a pediatrician can also provide antenatal care and support in the form of important education to the mother. A pediatrician can also guide the mother about necessary immunizations to prevent the passage of any infection to the fetus. A pediatric team will be present at the time of birth.

The role of the pediatrician at the time of childbirth is:

- To assess the physical health, breathing, and heart rate of the newborn.
- To assess the fetus for any injury that occurred during the delivery
- To evaluate the child of an infected mother for that infection
- To analyze the child of a diabetic mother for blood sugar levels
- To diagnose the fetus for any pathology and treat it accordingly
- To guide the mother on breastfeeding and immunizations.

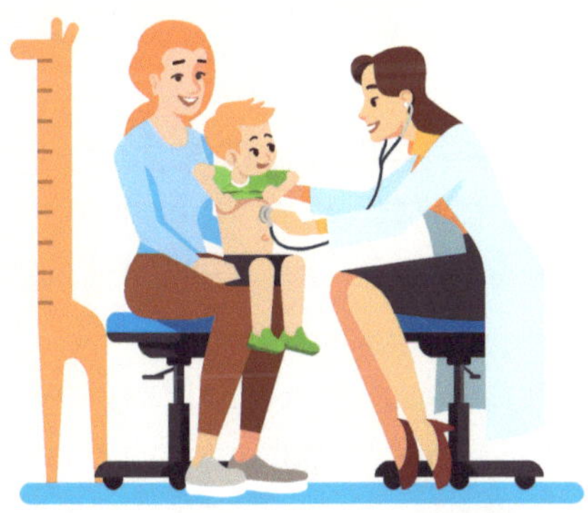

YOUR PREGNANCY AND DELIVERY TEAM

Specialists according to your medical history

If you have a history of a specific medical condition, assistance from the relevant medical specialist is necessary throughout the pregnancy to help prevent any complications for the mother and her child.

Benefits of a doula

Generally, a doula is a non-medical companion who is trained to assist and support you in various ways during labor and delivery. Doulas have varying backgrounds and you may find that some may have some clinical training before becoming a doula. A doula benefits you in the following ways:

- Provides emotional support through motivation and reassurance
- Informs you about certain procedures and provides some clarity on what is going on
- Can provide you with pain relief through massage and other techniques
- Informs you about the baby after delivery
- Helps you in the breastfeeding process after birth
- Serves as a medical advocate

Make sure to meet your doula well in advance of your delivery day

BONUS NUTRITION PLAN

To receive a free guide for a conception diet, simply send an email with the title: EBOOK MEAL-PLAN to info@visionarywomenshealth.com

Be sure to include your:
- Full Name
- Email Address (this must match your ebook order)

You will receive an email notification with your very own nutrition app where you will receive full meal plans, recipes, and grocery lists from Dr. Gueye as a thank you for reading this ebook to the end!

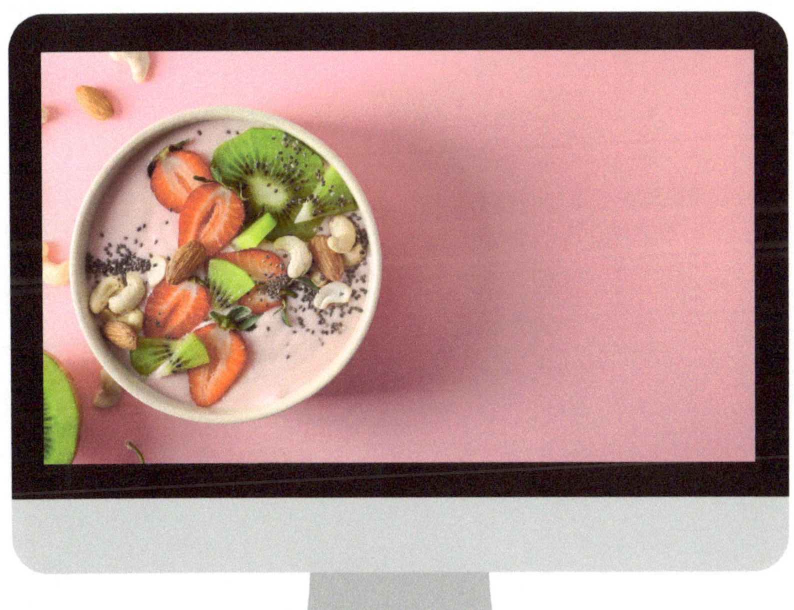

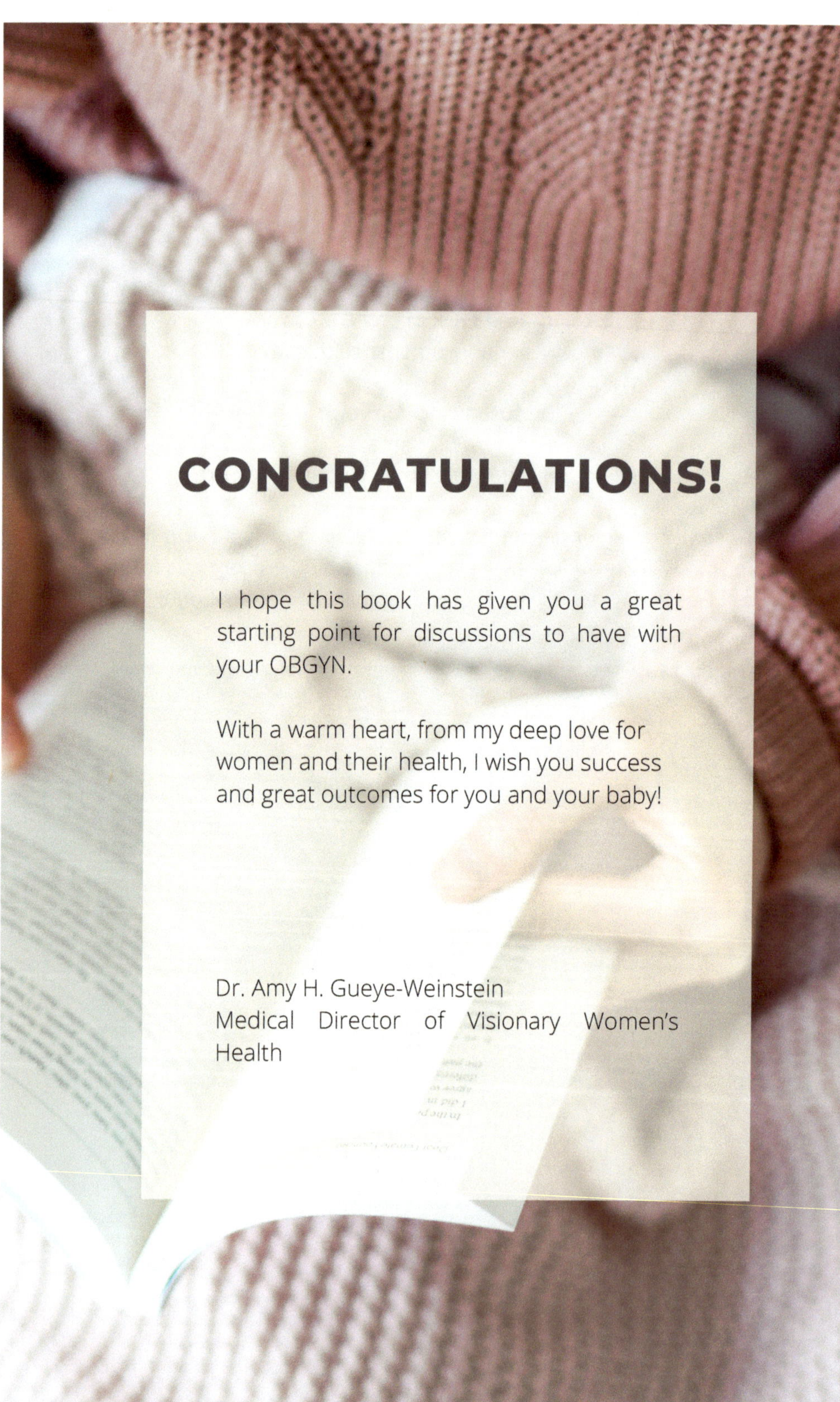
CONGRATULATIONS!

I hope this book has given you a great starting point for discussions to have with your OBGYN.

With a warm heart, from my deep love for women and their health, I wish you success and great outcomes for you and your baby!

Dr. Amy H. Gueye-Weinstein
Medical Director of Visionary Women's Health

www.ingramcontent.com/pod-product-compliance
Lightning Source LLC
Chambersburg PA
CBHW040230240726
48664CB00001B/75